The Glaucoma Screening Manual

The Glaucoma Screening Manual

Shibal Bhartiya
MBBS MS (Ophthalmology)
Senior Consultant
Department of Ophthalmology
Fortis Memorial Research Institute
Gurugram, Haryana, India

Foreword
Tanuj Dada

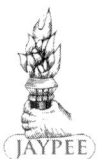

JAYPEE BROTHERS MEDICAL PUBLISHERS
The Health Sciences Publisher
New Delhi | London

Jaypee Brothers Medical Publishers (P) Ltd

Headquarters

Jaypee Brothers Medical Publishers (P) Ltd
EMCA House, 23/23-B
Ansari Road, Daryaganj
New Delhi 110 002, India
Landline: +91-11-23272143, +91-11-23272703
+91-11-23282021, +91-11-23245672
Email: jaypee@jaypeebrothers.com

Corporate Office

Jaypee Brothers Medical Publishers (P) Ltd
4838/24, Ansari Road, Daryaganj
New Delhi 110 002, India
Phone: +91-11-43574357
Fax: +91-11-43574314
Email: jaypee@jaypeebrothers.com

Overseas Office

JP Medical Ltd
83 Victoria Street, London
SW1H 0HW (UK)
Phone: +44 20 3170 8910
Fax: +44 (0)20 3008 6180
Email: info@jpmedpub.com

Website: www.jaypeebrothers.com
Website: www.jaypeedigital.com

© 2022, Jaypee Brothers Medical Publishers

The views and opinions expressed in this book are solely those of the original contributor(s)/author(s) and do not necessarily represent those of editor(s) of the book.

All rights reserved. No part of this publication may be reproduced, stored or transmitted in any form or by any means, electronic, mechanical, photocopying, recording or otherwise, without the prior permission in writing of the publishers.

All brand names and product names used in this book are trade names, service marks, trademarks or registered trademarks of their respective owners. The publisher is not associated with any product or vendor mentioned in this book.

Medical knowledge and practice change constantly. This book is designed to provide accurate, authoritative information about the subject matter in question. However, readers are advised to check the most current information available on procedures included and check information from the manufacturer of each product to be administered, to verify the recommended dose, formula, method and duration of administration, adverse effects and contraindications. It is the responsibility of the practitioner to take all appropriate safety precautions. Neither the publisher nor the author(s)/editor(s) assume any liability for any injury and/or damage to persons or property arising from or related to use of material in this book.

This book is sold on the understanding that the publisher is not engaged in providing professional medical services. If such advice or services are required, the services of a competent medical professional should be sought.

Every effort has been made where necessary to contact holders of copyright to obtain permission to reproduce copyright material. If any have been inadvertently overlooked, the publisher will be pleased to make the necessary arrangements at the first opportunity. The **CD/DVD-ROM** (if any) provided in the sealed envelope with this book is complimentary and free of cost. **Not meant for sale**.

Inquiries for bulk sales may be solicited at: jaypee@jaypeebrothers.com

The Glaucoma Screening Manual

First Edition: **2022**

ISBN: 978-93-5465-221-9

Printed at: Replika Press Pvt. Ltd.

Dedicated to
*Aradhya, and the children of the
Vision Unlimited After School Club*

Foreword

Glaucoma is the leading cause of blindness worldwide and 70-90% of cases remain undetected in the community in developing countries like India. Early detection of glaucoma is of vital importance as appropriate treatment can prevent blindness if done at the right time. In this regard, screening for glaucoma is critical and an unmet need in our healthcare systems.

The current practical manual by Dr Shibal Bhartiya, a globally renowned glaucoma specialist, gives a valuable insight into the logistics of setting up a screening facility.

The text includes details of the equipment, manpower, infrastructure required, community participation, publicity and valuable insights into data recording and action to be taken once screening is positive.

I hope *The Glaucoma Screening Manual* will ultimately help in detection of glaucoma in the community and be a critical step towards preventing blindness from glaucoma.

Tanuj Dada MBBS MD
Professor
Dr R P Centre for Ophthalmic Sciences
All India Institute of Medical Sciences
New Delhi, India

Preface

The Glaucoma Screening Manual is designed to be used by all healthcare professionals involved in glaucoma management, including nurses and allied healthcare professionals, and not just medical practitioners. Those planning to embark on community ophthalmology should find the book a valuable introduction to the diverse and unique challenges of this domain, and also to their varied and often, simple, solutions.

Practicing community ophthalmologists and allied healthcare practitioners must know how to communicate effectively, structure information, ask questions, and make robust clinical decisions, all in surroundings unfamiliar, and often, suboptimal. Working in screening programs often is a test of will power, as much as clinical decision-making, and this manual hopes to provide the tools that can be the foundation for both.

An evaluative framework is critical to assessing the feasibility of any screening program, and it has been my endeavor to stick to basic principles and common sense as the organizing structure, including information with, hopefully, a long half-life. And it is my sincere hope that the lucidity of this text makes up for any limitations in its comprehensiveness.

Best wishes, always.

Shibal Bhartiya

Acknowledgments

This book derives from my own experiences in community service as the Founder of Vision Unlimited, and from those of many expert colleagues, Drs Tanuj Dada, Tarek M Shaarawy and Parul Ichhpujani have helped me in sourcing, writing and structuring what is written, and what I practice each day. Dr Parul Ichhpujani, also one of my dearest friends, has helped with proofreading and the inevitable "I cannot believe you forgot that".

Nikhil has, as always, gone through my writing with a machete, deleting adjectives and adverbs and all turns of phrase deemed irrelevant and incomprehensible. Grashmi, is a partner in all that Vision Unlimited envisions, and endeavors to do, and so many of the learning in this book are our shared experiences.

And, of course, there is Aradhya, the reason why everything seems easy and worthwhile.

I would like to thank Shri Jitendar P Vij (Group Chairman), Mr Ankit Vij (Managing Director), and Ms Chetna Malhotra Vohra (Associate Director-Content Strategy) of M/s Jaypee Brothers Medical Publishers (P) Ltd, New Delhi, India, for their untiring support and encouragement. This book seeing the light of day is definitely also a testimony to their patience with my inability to comprehend deadlines.

To all of you, my love, and gratitude always.

Contents

1. **Screening: The Rationale and Feasibility** 1
   - Criteria for Positive Screen *2*
   - Lacunae *6*
   - Feasibility of Screening *7*

2. **Whom to Screen** 8
   - Community-based Screening *8*
   - Opportunistic Screening *8*

3. **Location of Screening Activity** 9

4. **Program Management Timelines** 10
   - Phase 1: Manpower Planning *10*
   - Phase 2: Prescreening Protocol Implementation *10*
   - Phase 3: Screening Day *11*
   - Phase 4: Monitoring and Reporting *11*

5. **Conforming with Regulation** 12
   - General Guidelines for Seeking Permissions *12*
   - General Guidelines for Ethical Clinical Practice *13*

6. **Prescreening Protocol** 15

7. **Information, Education and Communication** 18
   - Mass Approach *18*
   - Group Approach *19*
   - Individual Approach *20*
   - IEC Material *20*

8. **The Team** 23
   - Essential *23*
   - Desirable *24*

9. Community Participation 26
- Voluntary Organizations *26*
- Local Medical Practitioners *26*
- Non-Governmental Organizations (NGO) *26*
- Organizations/Associations *27*
- Government Sector *27*
- Media *27*

10. Equipment Checklist 28
- Registration Station *28*
- Visual Acuity Station *28*
- Tonometry Station *28*
- Slit-lamp Station *28*
- Counselor Station (Optional) *29*
- Emergency Medication Kit *29*
- Miscellaneous *30*

11. On Site Checklist 31
- Furniture *31*
- Electrical Points *31*
- Hygiene Facilities *31*
- Adequate Emergency Exits *32*

12. Patient Flow 33

13. Standard Operating Procedures 34
- Visual Acuity *34*
- Non-contact Tonometry *36*
- Anterior Chamber Depth *37*
- Slit-lamp Biomicroscopy: Fundus Examination 90 D Lens *39*
- Goldmann Applanation Tonometry *40*
- Gonioscopy *42*

14. Postscreening Follow-up 44

15. Efficacy Measures 46
- Efficacy Measures for the Screening Program *46*
- Performance Parameters to be Evaluated for Each of the Screening Units *47*
- Supervisors *47*
- Timelines *48*

Appendix 49
- Waiver *49*
- Screening Form *51*
- Postscreening Form *53*
- Screening Feedback Form *54*

Index *55*

CHAPTER 1

Screening: The Rationale and Feasibility

The cost-effectiveness of general population screening for glaucoma has not been clearly established and there is no consensus in current available literature regarding the timing or frequency of population screening. This has been variably attributed to lack of suitability of available tests, the low prevalence of the disease, and the questionable effectiveness of early treatment.

There is consensus that targeted screening of individuals at risk of glaucoma may be warranted, and may be more cost-effective in specific subgroups of the population such as older adults, African descent populations, and those with a family history of glaucoma. However, the cut-off level of glaucoma prevalence needed to make screening desirable is not known. Also, there is increasing stress on the importance of screening for open-angle glaucoma because patients remain asymptomatic until late in disease progression, when visual loss and functional impairment are irreversible. Amongst Asians, angle closure has been identified to be far more common than believed earlier. Also, since the intervention (laser peripheral iridotomy) is a one time procedure, its impact on preventing blindness is far more.

The ideal test for screening would be one which is low cost, reproducible, with high specificity (few false positives) and sensitivity (low false negatives).

At present, there is no single test that provides a reasonable balance of sensitivity and specificity for detecting early glaucoma. Sensitivity can be increased by combining tests and defining a positive screen as either test meeting the criterion of positivity. This, however, results in a concomitant loss of specificity, and consequently cost-effectiveness.

A screening program includes defining the population, identifying conditions to screen, determining a test protocol, marketing and recruitment, follow through, and efficacy measures.

CRITERIA FOR POSITIVE SCREEN

The following criteria may be taken as a positive screen:
- Non-contact tonometry >21
- *Anterior segment examination:* Van Herick test, lens status
- *Slit-lamp biomicroscopy:* Cup:Disc ratio > 0.6, cup asymmetry > 0.2, neuroretinal rim (NRR) pattern and disc hemorrhages.
- Van Herick grade 1-2

The rationale for the protocol design is as follows:

Tonometry

Tonometry has been popular as a glaucoma screening test, but it is now universally accepted that no intraocular pressure criterion of positivity provides an acceptable balance of sensitivity and specificity. Data from the Baltimore Eye Survey showed that if an intraocular pressure value of 21 mm Hg or higher is used, the sensitivity would be only 47.1%, with a specificity of 92.4%. If the intraocular pressure value for positivity is lowered, sensitivity increases,

Screening: The Rationale and Feasibility

but the specificity lowers to such an extent that it is only 65% at a cut-off value of 19 mm Hg or higher. For our screening protocol, in order to not overload the screening machinery with high false positives, the IOP threshold is taken to be >21 mm Hg. A Goldmann Applanation Tonometry should be performed on each of the subjects with non-contact tonometer (NCT) >21 mm Hg.

An evaluation of the relative merits of tonometry for pooled all stages of glaucoma revealed that:

Tonometer	Sensitivity (CI 95%)	Specificity (CI 95%)	DOR (CI 95%)
Goldmann Applanation	46 (22–71)	95 (89–97)	4.95 (4.48–48.95)
Non-contact Airpuff Tonometer	92 (62–100)	92 (90–94)	134.88 (17.15–1061.1)

(DOR: diagnostic odds ratio)

Given the acceptable operating characteristics of the NCT, ease of use and decreased risk of transmission of infections, the NCT remains the tool of choice for screening for elevated IOP.

Note: The Perkins applanation tonometer is a portable, handheld device that works on the same principle as the Goldmann Applanation Tonometer. It is especially useful in patients who are obese, bedridden, or difficult to position on the slit lamp.

The Icare TA01i uses the principle of rebound tonometry, and provides a simple, rapid, reliable, and accurate measurement of IOP. It may be useful as a handheld screening tool instead of the NCT since unlike GAT, it does not require the use of anesthesia, and is relatively easier to perform. The device probe may be sterilized between patients using isopropranolol.

Slit-lamp Anterior Segment Biomicroscopy

Anterior segment biomicroscopy is useful for identifying the risks of angle closure such as the depth of central and peripheral anterior chamber, contour of iris (e.g., bombe) as well as previous attacks of angle closure. These include sectoral iris atrophy, glaukomflecken, posterior synechiae and peripheral anterior synechiae. Signs of secondary glaucoma causes, such as features of uveitis, pigment dispersion (iris transillumination and pigment deposits on the corneal endothelium), pseudoexfoliation (on lens capsule), iris rubeosis (neovascular causes), can also be identified. Measuring limbal ACD (modified van Herick test) appears the most promising, as it can help detect all stages of primary angle-closure disease due to pupil block and nonpupil block.

It is critical to remember that the van Herick test misses a substantial proportion of angle closure while incorrectly identifying roughly 1 in 8 open-angle eyes as closed.

All patients with shallow peripheral anterior chambers (van Herick Grade 0, 1, or 2) must undergo a gonioscopy with a four mirror lens, to ascertain both, angle anatomy, and, to differentiate between appositional and synechial closure.

Optic Nerve Head Assessment

Optic nerve assessment with ophthalmoscopy also suffers from poor sensitivity and specificity. Additional drawbacks include the need for highly trained examiners, the wide variability in agreement in the assessment of optic nerve status, and the need to dilate the pupils to allow adequate visualization. Direct ophthalmoscopy has a reported sensitivity of 59% and a specificity of 73% in detecting and classifying optic disc changes associated with glaucoma, and is recommended following dilation of pupils. Given the poor specificity and sensitivity of the test, and the fact that dilation is a time consuming process which may not be acceptable to the patient, a slit-lamp biomicroscopic assessment of the optic disc using a 90 D fundus lens must be performed, noting the following parameters: Increased cupping of the optic nerve head, asymmetry in the amount of cupping between eyes, neuroretinal rim pattern, and optic disc hemorrhages.

In case of diabetics and cases with suspected retinal pathologies, a decision may be taken by the ophthalmologist to perform a dilated fundus examination. However, it is imperative that narrow angles be ruled out (van Herick Grade 3 and 4 only), prior to mydriasis.

The use of Artificial Intelligence (AI) based on deep learning applied to non-mydriatic ONH photographs has sparked tremendous global interest in recent years. AI, in conjunction with telemedicine, has the potential to revolutionize not only screening, but also the diagnosis and monitoring of major eye diseases, including glaucoma.

Numerous AI strategies have been shown to elicit acceptable specificity and sensitivity for structural (optical coherence tomography imaging, fundus photography) and functional (visual field testing) tests. As is true for clinical practice, a combination of structural and functional inputs improves the diagnostic ability.

AI algorithms, therefore, may enhance the efficiency, productivity, and quality of the screening program.

However, to date, there is no externally validated algorithm for glaucoma screening, and the transition from "black box" to "explainable AI," is essential before its widespread use. However, given the successful adoption of AI strategies for diabetic retinopathy and retinopathy of prematurity screening programs, it is clear that AI will inevitably shape the future of glaucoma screening, as well as its management.

It is therefore prudent to consider one of the two, either non-mydriatic fundus camera photos, or smartphone-based fundus photography, as part of screening protocols.

Visual Acuity

Since visual acuity is an independent risk factor for decreased vision-related quality of life, and contributes significantly to impaired performance of everyday tasks of living, the vision must be tested for each of the screened subjects.

LACUNAE

Even though disc and nerve fiber layer evaluation, or both, using image devices may increase sensitivity, specificity, and nerve fiber layer evaluation, or both, using imaging devices may increase sensitivity, specificity, and reproducibility, these techniques are resource intensive and not practical for mass screenings.

Similarly, even though functional tests namely, perimetry, are fast gaining acceptance for screening, their use is beyond the scope of most screening protocols.

Their moderately poor specificity, expense, the amount of time necessary for testing, and the relative lack of portability of most of the available perimeters pose limitations for the screening setting. Of the available technologies, the Melbourne Rapid Fields is the most promising as a screening tool. It requires minimal human contact and can be easily sanitized in under two minutes, thereby mitigating the risk of cross contamination between patients. The convenient easy-to-use software offers rapid testing on Apple iPads (generation 3/4 and later) and online on laptop and desktop PC screens via cloud.

Recent advances in technology have provided anterior segment topography systems which provide the opportunity to analyze the anterior segment of the eye in a non-contact manner. However, they do not provide the details of signs of past angle closure, recession, peripheral anterior synechiae or physical patency of the angle. They are also expensive with a relative lack of portability, and are a poor substitute for gonioscopy.

FEASIBILITY OF SCREENING

The determinants of the predictive value of a given screening test are its sensitivity and specificity, along with the prevalence of asymptomatic disease in the population. Since no statistics regarding prevalence of glaucoma are available for the population to be screened, a predictive value for even the most valid test cannot be ascertained. Most screening protocols are designed to get the most at-risk for glaucoma population within the purview of the available medical care.

Any population-based screening program aims to operate on two tiers: (1) It increases the awareness about the disease with the local population, thus potentially increasing case detection and (2) It increases the positive screen to case conversion in the secondary/tertiary care centers during the second phase of opportunistic screening of those patients who are identified as high-risk from population screenings.

CHAPTER 2

Whom to Screen

COMMUNITY-BASED SCREENING

- All subjects presenting for screening
- *All subjects:* Caucasians over the age of 50, and for those of Asian or African descent, age over 40.
- All first-degree relatives of glaucoma patients, commencing 5–10 years earlier than the age of onset of glaucoma in their affected relative.
- Individuals with myopia, abnormal blood pressure, history of migraine, diabetes, peripheral vasospasm, eye injury and history of/ongoing steroid use.

Special Attention Related to Primary Angle Closure Disease (PACD)

Individuals with hypermetropia, family history of angle closure, advancing age, female gender, Asian or Inuit descent and shallow anterior chamber.

This is of critical importance in the Indian scenario, where almost half of the patients of glaucoma have angle closure.

OPPORTUNISTIC SCREENING

- Diabetes clinics/Geriatric clinics
- Old age homes
- First-degree relatives of glaucoma patients
- Cataract patients attending general clinics

CHAPTER 3

Location of Screening Activity

To decide where to hold the screening program, it is important to remember that the location changes depending on the methodology. In context, since both community outreach and opportunistic screening are envisaged as part of any screening protocol, the following are the criteria for each arm of the screening program.

When choosing a location for the eye camp in the community, the following must be kept in mind:

- *Ease of access:* The site should be accessible by public transport.
- *Acceptable:* To all members of the community.
- *Area:* For a camp with an expected turn out of 300, the minimum requirement is two rooms of width at least 7 m or 25 feet for checking vision. In case the maximum room width is less than 7 m, the E-chart reflected with a mirror may be used at 3 m. It must have a separate waiting area for patients.
- The available options could be schools, community halls, places of worship, etc.
- Whenever possible, community should be encouraged to provide the space.

For opportunistic screening the following are possible locations:
- Diabetic clinics
- Geriatric clinics
- Old age homes

CHAPTER 4: Program Management Timelines

Before the screening program is scheduled, it is important that the timelines for the ancillary activities critical for its success are clearly established.

PHASE 1: MANPOWER PLANNING

Each screening unit must do an individual, best-fit manpower planning depending on available resources and expected turn out for the screening program. Recruitment and selection the members of the project team at the implementing center is to be carried out in consultation with the appropriate authorities. The training schedule for the field staff can be framed according to the different cadres of the project. However, it is advisable to have a common orientation workshop/training session for the entire team. Screening techniques and standardization of examination methods are key and should be carried out meticulously not just for the support staff but also for certified ophthalmologists and residents in training.

PHASE 2: PRESCREENING PROTOCOL IMPLEMENTATION

Distribution of materials for information, education and communication should commence at least 2 weeks before the scheduled day of screening. All possible methods of mass and group approach must be implemented in order to publicize the date and location of the screening camp.

PHASE 3: SCREENING DAY

The screening is to be carried out on the specified day, at the specified location in accordance to the screening protocol. All standard operating procedures and referral end points are to be strictly adhered to. Any deviations from the protocol must be noted, and duly justified.

PHASE 4: MONITORING AND REPORTING

Each screening day data is to be reviewed by the team leader within a week of the screening day and duly dispatched to the nodal agency responsible for data collection. Review of postscreening follow-up must be made within the appropriate time points (2-6 weeks postscreening). The relevant data from the follow-up must be dispatched to the nodal agency within 8 weeks of screening day.

Quarterly review meetings or teleconferencing may be organized with the members of the senior management team, together with the heads of the project, whenever feasible, for each of the regions.

The interim analysis should be scheduled for 12 months from institution of the screening program and final analysis at the end of 24 months, to ascertain its impact.

CHAPTER 5

Conforming with Regulation

Given that this protocol is designed for application in several countries, with different community health regulations, and hopes to involve individuals from both public and private institutions, individual team leaders have to be responsible for obtaining the requisite permissions from the appropriate authorities.

GENERAL GUIDELINES FOR SEEKING PERMISSIONS

The general guidelines for seeking required permissions are outlined below, as a reference:

- The participating doctors/healthcare practitioners must obtain permission from suitable authorities for participation in the screening program. Involving senior colleagues, residents and fellows, as well as medical/nursing students will strengthen the screening program and help create a generation sensitized to the need for vigilance against glaucoma.
- In case of healthcare professionals working in the public healthcare system, all efforts must be made to get written permission from the appropriate governmental agency.
- The possibility of considering the screening program as "on duty" in terms of either financial remuneration or a compensatory off must be discussed with the employers/nodal agency.

- Permission and support of the local administration and local administrative authorities must be sought for the specified duration, and location of screening. Inviting elected representatives to participate in the program is a good public relations exercise.
- Community participation results in better acceptability and increased recruitment. It also is very effective in removing several hurdles that may crop up in the course of planning the screening exercise.

GENERAL GUIDELINES FOR ETHICAL CLINICAL PRACTICE

The general guidelines of ethical clinical practice are outlined below, as a reference:

- Screening for all individuals seeking medical attention, regardless of gender, faith, belief, racial, or political affiliations.
- Results of the screening, whether positive or negative will be explained to the patient keeping in mind the quality of life impact of a positive screen, and the false sense of security that a negative screen may induce.
- Each individual must be advised that the screening is not a substitute for a comprehensive eye examination, and does not imply protection from other diseases.
- All efforts must be made to facilitate the process of further examination of positive screens in secondary/tertiary care centers, ensuring that those diagnosed have access to treatment and all attempts must be made to monitor and ensure compliance.
- All ocular emergencies must be attended to, with available resources on the spot, before referral to the nearest ophthalmic center for further management.

- All first-degree relatives of known glaucoma patients and suspects must be screened by actively soliciting their participation.
- The examining doctor should remember, however, that this protocol is guidance, and not a substitute for clinical acumen. If the practitioner is confident that disease has not been excluded (in spite of no documented evidence), it is reasonable to continue to refer the patient for subsequent examinations, and vice versa.
- Consent for participation in screening is implied by a person seeking it. However, a verbal consent must be sought (either from that person if he or she has the capacity to consent, or from the person's guardian or any person or organization authorized by law) before any contact procedures, after explaining the process to the patient. Each patient must sign a waiver at the time of registration in duplicate, and a copy of the same must be filed with the screening team along with the screening proforma.

CHAPTER 6

Prescreening Protocol

There is consensus that conducting population-based mass screenings for glaucoma is expensive, largely inaccurate and places a burden on the healthcare system which is not entirely cost-effective. Opportunistic screening alone, however, does not cater to the needs of population with asymptomatic disease since access to health care as well as awareness are often lacking.

Even though recent studies have shown that conducting self- recruited population screenings by advertising about the risks and symptoms of glaucoma are also not effective, a prescreening awareness campaign has a dual impact. It results in awareness about the disease, and the fact that a healthcare resource is available at a particular point in time, within easy access, free of cost. It also results in a quantum of self-selection at the population level, thereby targeting the at-risk group. Combining glaucoma screening programs with screening for cataract and diabetic retinopathy can make it more cost-effective.

The screening protocol envisages the following as a prescreening awareness campaign:

- Involving the community for dissemination of information regarding location and time of screening camp: Whenever applicable, Resident Welfare Associations, local key opinion leaders, school teachers, local officials and people's representatives should be contacted for support. The use of banners, posters, pamphlets and

announcements during communal prayers should be encouraged.
- Community participation by way of infrastructural support should be solicited in terms of providing the space where the screening is conducted. Mosques, temples, churches community halls, schools, private courtyards/halls are potential locations for the camp. Volunteers to help with organization from within the community should be welcomed and allocated tasks visible to the community like registration. Volunteers should not be encouraged to participate in the critical steps of the screening protocol, which must all be carried out by the visiting doctor and paramedical workers.
- In anticipation of the one-day screening clinics, the week prior to the screening camp, local organizers should to be recruited and invited for discussion and education about the objectives of the clinic. These organizers must in turn, to be responsible for helping with advertising for the camp (e.g., through posters, flyers, or door-to-door visits), managing volunteers, and managing the patient influx.
- Given the widespread use of smartphones, even in remote areas, the use of Whatsapp and SMSs can revolutionize the reach of the IEC program.
- Public glaucoma educational sessions, whenever possible, using mass media such as the local radio and television channels, as well as social media, should be used to reach the target group.
- The message for publicity must be tailored to local needs. But the key points to be emphasized include:
  - Glaucoma is asymptomatic and potentially blinding
  - Early diagnosis results in preservation of vision

- *High-risk group:* Trauma, steroids, use of glasses, family history of glaucoma
- Screening program by well-qualified medical practitioner
- Near your home, free of cost

- *Glaucoma Awareness Week:* A regional glaucoma awareness week, not necessarily co-incident with the World Glaucoma Week may be determined depending on local weather conditions, public holidays and feasts. This celebration can be part of the prescreening awareness campaign, geared towards generating public interest and awareness regarding the burden of disease, its asymptomatic nature and the recognition of at-risk groups.
- Planned advertising with an appropriate lead time of 2 weeks, targeting the local population by means of mass media, social media, banners and door-to-door campaigns.
- Additional human resources can be made available through organizations which may include: Non-Governmental Organizations (NGO), Lions Club, Rotary Clubs, Student Federations, religious missions with focus on health or education, public health clinics, community health centers, or university affiliated clinics that provide free or discounted care. Networking with a coalition of like-minded groups may result in increased manpower availability, better publicity and consequently, a more dynamic community response.
- All campaign, publicity material and patient information brochures must be made available in at least two languages: Local language and English, in most areas, to ensure maximum outreach. Resource material may be adapted from: http://www.eugs.org/eng-paz/default.asp.

CHAPTER 7

Information, Education and Communication

Information, education and communication (IEC) implies sharing information and ideas in a way that is culturally acceptable to the community by using appropriate channels, messages, and methods. It is one of the most important tools in health promotion and community mobilization, and has the potential to modify community behavior.

The generic guidelines for development of glaucoma awareness messages are mentioned below, and will need minor modifications to suit regional needs:
- Messages should be tailored for cultural acceptability, literacy levels, available infrastructure, and to the specific target audience, and may be delivered by a variety of channels in different forms.
- The message must be simple, concise, and relevant to the target audience. It is essential that the language used is objective, unbiased and consistent, as well as being directly linked to service delivery.

The three broad categories of strategies for creating awareness vary in terms of method of delivery and target audience, and are described below.

MASS APPROACH

The mass approach aims to create general awareness and knowledge of a topic or event in a particular community; in context, about glaucoma the disease, as also the screening initiative. Tools for this include press meetings, radio and television (audio messages reaching the visually impaired), banners and posters in hospitals and public meeting places. Pamphlets and booklets about glaucoma, and the screening program may be distributed. Mike announcements about location and timing of screening may also turn-out.

Whatsapp messages and bulk SMSs can reach target audience, and reminders can be sent on the day of the planned screening as well, to increase participation. Also, dissemination of information about at-risk cases will mean an increased response from the target population. Trade exhibitions, local fairs, and prayer meetings provide a unique opportunity to reach a large audience through the use of a booth distributing IEC materials while providing a forum for interaction between screening staff and the public.

GROUP APPROACH

The group approach targets smaller audiences, and aims to add to the awareness and knowledge, over a sustained period of time. A modification of attitudes, conceptions, and practice patterns is also envisaged through this, assuming that the audience already possesses some level of awareness and some form of basic knowledge of the problem. In context, a continuing medical education (CME) program to sensitize healthcare providers towards the need for vigilance for glaucoma, and adoption of practices like intraocular pressure measurements by optometrists and paramedical personnel and referral to higher centers of at-risk individuals. The tools used include guest lectures, group discussions and provision of resource materials such as videos and hands-on training sessions. In context, these may be conducted during orientation training for the screening team, teachers' meetings, religious gatherings, and patient support group meetings, etc.

INDIVIDUAL APPROACH

Individual approach or individual counseling is targeted at the individual, and is the most effective in influencing knowledge, attitudes, and behavior. A one-on-one interaction means tailoring of the information to best fit the needs of the individual, keeping in mind his/her relevant requirements, limitations and patterns of health-seeking behavior. The exercise aims to alter any incorrect perceptions concerning glaucoma.

Although this approach has the greatest possibility of success, it is resource intensive; and it is conducted only after mass and group campaigns.

Counseling aims to establish a relationship of trust between patient and healthcare worker, empowering the patient to make realistic, logical decisions and act on it.

IEC MATERIAL

Posters are intended to raise general awareness in the community about the problem of glaucoma and should be placed in visible locations, frequented by the target audience, e.g., diabetes clinics, waiting rooms in hospitals, optical shops, medical shops, local meeting places, and bus stops.

Booklets/brochures aimed at educating medical practitioners and paramedical personnel on the subject of glaucoma and its management have to be designed and distributed.

Pamphlets are an ideal way to educate glaucoma suspects and patients about the nature and implications of glaucoma, and encourage health-seeking behavior.

All these may be distributed physically, and as PDFs or images on social media.

Teaching slides and videos are extremely useful in disseminating information, as they facilitate educational sessions, allowing graphical illustrations of otherwise complicated medical information.

Attractive infographics sent via social media channels, especially Whatsapp and TikTok have widespread appeal and retention value.

The training components are to be modified from one screening unit to another. Each of the team members, however, needs to be briefed about the screening protocol, questionnaire and the standard operating procedures. A rational curriculum development and creation of teaching materials must be tailored to the particular community.

Publicity material should contain information on where, when, for what, and to whom these camps are useful. Moreover, as the target group is in the economically active age group (or older, and consequently dependent for transport) there should be a lead time of at least 2 weeks between the start of promotional activities and the camp.

The organizers may refer to:
1. The European Glaucoma Society guidelines regarding patient education material available as a free online resource at http://www.eugs.org/eng-paz/default.asp.
2. The World Glaucoma Association statement on screening for glaucoma available as a free online resource at https://wga.one/wga/screening-for-open-angle-glaucoma/.

3. Other useful online resources include:
   - https://www.glaucoma.org
   - https://www.glaucomapatients.org
   - https://visionaware.org/get-connected/about-visionaware/glaucoma/
   - https://www.brightfocus.org/glaucoma.

CHAPTER 8

The Team

Individual units must be customized for each of the screening camps. The minimum acceptable team strength is one member each from groups 1 and 3, and at least two from group 2.

ESSENTIAL

- *Ophthalmologist(s):* After having attended basic resource training, the doctor in charge of the screening protocol should be given a certification of eligibility in conducting the screening procedure as per the protocol design.
- *Nurse/Paramedical worker (PMW):* After having attended a basic resource training in recording visual acuity, NCT, and administering the questionnaire; the nurse/PMW should be given a certification of eligibility in carrying out visual acuity testing and NCT as per the protocol design.
- *Volunteer/Medical student:* After having attended a basic resource training in sensitization to the protocol design and objectives and administering the questionnaire, the volunteer/medical student may be considered eligible to act as facilitator during the screening process, aiding with registration and patient flow.

DESIRABLE

- *Counselor:* Preferably a local resident of the healthcare team, with superior communication skills, well conversant with the socioeconomic problems of the population screened should be sensitized to the screening protocol. The counselor will be responsible for:
  - *Communicating to the patient the implications of a positive screen:* "It does not mean you have the disease, but the probability of you having the disease is high, so further investigations are mandatory."
  - *Communicating to the patient the implications of a negative screen:* "Chances that you have this disease are negligible at this time, but you may develop the disease, or other eye problems, at a later date. Annual eye examinations are mandatory. Screening is not a substitute for a comprehensive eye examination"
  - *Postscreening follow-up:* Ensuring that each positive screen must have a definitive examination to diagnose glaucoma; and in case of diagnosis be entered into care, and persist in receiving care. First-degree relatives of each newly diagnosed case must be invited to undergo the definitive examination to rule out glaucoma.
  - *Facilitating further communication between the community and the screening program:* To facilitate an ongoing dialogue and patient care so as to establish a long term relationship, thereby ensuring success of subsequent screening programs, and longitudinal follow-ups.

- *Team leader:* A member of the healthcare team with the zeal and vision necessary to keep the team together and motivated. The team leader is responsible for:
    - On the spot problem solving, dealing with conflicts within the team and outside in a manner acceptable to all
    - Managing time schedules and shifts, also resource and personnel allocation, depending on the needs of the particular camp
    - Supervising prescreening and postscreening activities, locating and correcting lacunae in communication
    - Coordinating with local authorities regarding regulatory issues, obtaining permissions from the competent authorities for organizing the camp
    - Liaison with NGO, local volunteer groups, clubs and student bodies to enlist support for the awareness campaigns and organizational logistics.

In case manpower resources do not permit recruitment of counselors and team leaders, the screening team members are expected to take over their roles.

CHAPTER 9

Community Participation

Community participation is key to the success of any screening program and the following organizations may provide key resources in terms of manpower and organizational skills.

VOLUNTARY ORGANIZATIONS

Voluntary organizations are recognized by the community as providers of care, and have a systematic plan and strategy to reach the community in place already. Collaboration with these organizations thereby increases the impact of the screening program.

LOCAL MEDICAL PRACTITIONERS

Local medical practitioners are recognized as healthcare providers and therefore, can greatly influence participation by encouraging self-enrolment and referrals from their own practice.

NON-GOVERNMENTAL ORGANIZATIONS (NGO)

They are working at the grassroots level and are conversant with the specific needs and schedules of the particular community. They also have strong networks and organizational skills.

ORGANIZATIONS/ASSOCIATIONS

Organizations/associations (youth, religious) are usually groups of highly motivated individuals with a strong sense of commitment, and with emotional ties within the community. They can prove invaluable in terms of motivation and community mobilization.

GOVERNMENT SECTOR

It is a problem typical to the developing world that even though the chief functionaries of government agencies are committed to community-based screening programs, an actual one often meets with apathy. It is therefore advisable to interact with officials and elected representatives and secure their active participation.

MEDIA

The media is a key networking partner. Radio and television are invaluable for spreading information into rural areas and amongst illiterate populations. Newspaper articles and advertisements effectively spread information to those who read them.

The role of social media, including SMSs, Whatsapp, Twitter, Facebook and TikTok, cannot be overemphasized. With increasing smartphone usage and cheaper data plans, even the less privileged sections of the society can be reached effectively. It is definitely more cost-effective than mass media, and has the potential to revolutionize health-related IEC, if used appropriately.

CHAPTER 10

Equipment Checklist

REGISTRATION STATION

- Proforma
- Pens
- Measuring tape
- Scratch pads
- Referral sheets
- Register/Laptops/Computers for record keeping
- Patient education material including brochures, banners and posters

VISUAL ACUITY STATION

- Snellens/E-charts
- Tumbling E plastic prototype
- Pinhole
- Occluder
- Torch/Flashlight
- Autorefractometer (optional)

TONOMETRY STATION

Airpuff tonometer/Non-contact airpuff tonometer (NCT)/I-Care

SLIT-LAMP STATION

- Slit lamp
- 90/78 D lens

- Adaptor for smartphone photography/non-mydratic fundus camera
- Direct ophthalmoscope
- Goldmann applanation tonometer
- Gonioscope (four mirror)
- Fluorescien strips
- Local anesthetic
- Tissue paper
- Torch/Flashlight
- Antibiotic drops
- Rub-on disinfectant
- Cotton tipped applicators
- Alcohol swabs
- Gloves in different sizes

COUNSELOR STATION (OPTIONAL)

- Referral slips
- Directions to the hospital
- Business cards of doctors and optometrists
- Patient information brochures
- Computer (preferably with internet, to help set-up appointments for further investigations and management)

EMERGENCY MEDICATION KIT

- Acetazolamide tablets
- Antibiotic eye drops
- Timolol eye drops
- Prostaglandin analogue eye drops
- Steroid eye drops
- Mydriatic eye drops (Tropicamide and homatropine)

- First aid kit for trauma including sterile bandages, cotton, band-aids, swabs, betadine, and antibiotic ointment
- Emergency kit for medical emergencies, including BP instrument, stethoscope, etc.

MISCELLANEOUS

- Extension cords
- Surge protectors
- Spare bulbs for slit lamp

On Site Checklist

FURNITURE

- *Tables:* Six or more
- *Chairs:* Six or more
- *Stools:* Six or more
- Chairs/benches for patients in the waiting area
- *Equipment for maintaining ambient temperature:* Fans/coolers/heaters/air conditioners
- Laptops/computers for record keeping, printers
- Stationary including pens, registers, paper staplers, pins, and post-it notes

ELECTRICAL POINTS

- A minimum of two electric plug points per station
- *Adequate ambient light:* Natural + Artificial to enable visual acuity testing
- If possible, separate room for slit-lamp examination, preferably with low levels of ambient lighting

HYGIENE FACILITIES

- A minimum of two toilets, separate for men and women
- Drinking water, disposable plastic cups
- Food and refreshments for camp staff and volunteers
- Vehicles for transportation of eyecamp staff

ADEQUATE EMERGENCY EXITS

- Locations with separate entry and exits should be preferred. If not possible, areas to facilitate patient movement should be demarcated clearly.
- Evacuation exit plan must be formulated on site during setting-up the camp.

CHAPTER 12

Patient Flow

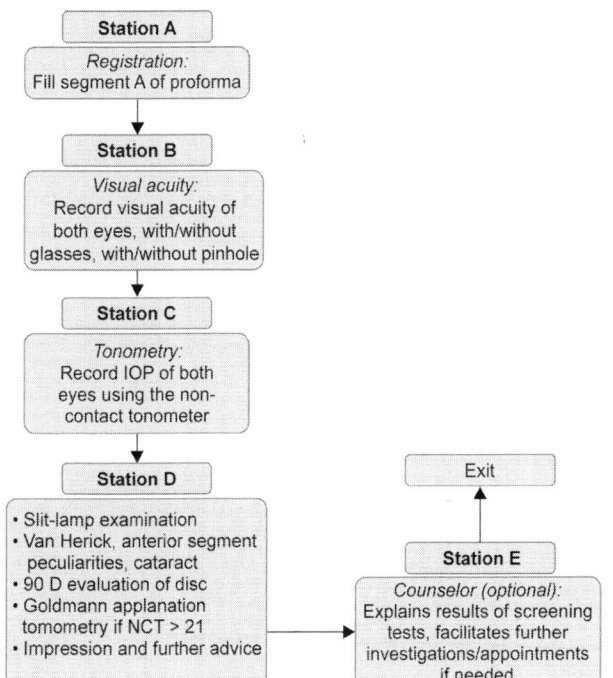

CHAPTER 13

Standard Operating Procedures

The following appendix is in addition to the training material which must be provided to the healthcare professionals before the commencement of the training program. It constitutes a ready reckoner to facilitate consistency in the performance of a specific function, critical to the screening protocol.

The patient, at the time of registration, must sign a waiver in duplicate, a copy of which should be provided to the patient. The screening proforma must also be duly filled in duplicate, one copy of which should be provided to the patient after counseling, and the other filed by the screening team.

VISUAL ACUITY

Indications: Routine examination

Materials: Snellen Visual Acuity Chart, Pinhole occluder

Method: Seat the patient comfortably at a distance of 6 meters (or 3 m), as measured using the measuring tape provided, from the Snellen chart, looking straight ahead in a well lit room. Ensure that there is no bright light reflecting off the chart.

Cover the patient's left eye with the occluder (*or* ask him/her to cover his/her left eye gently with his/her own palm), and ask him/her to read from the chart in front. If the person reads all the letters of one line correctly, but cannot read any of the letters of the next line, record vision as the Snellen fraction of the line that was read correctly. If the person reads all the letters of one line correctly, and some of the letters of the next line, record vision as the Snellen fraction of the line plus the number of letters of the next line that were read correctly.

In case the patient cannot read even the top line (VA < 6/60), hold up fingers for the patient to count at progressively distances of 3, 2 and 1 m. The farthest distance at which the patient can see and count fingers correctly is recorded as CF @ x meters (Counting Fingers at x meters).

In case the patient is unable to count fingers, wave your hand at a distance of 20 cm from the patient's face. In case the patient can perceive movement, record VA as HM (Hand Movements).

In case the patient is unable to see hand movements, check for perception of light. Shine a bright light in front of the patient's eye, at a distance of 20 cm. In case the patient can see the light, record VA as PL (Perception of Light). Shine the light from each of the four quadrants, (nasal, temporal, superior and inferior) and record in which of the quadrants the patient can correctly perceive the direction of light. Record the projection on an 'X' where each prong of the 'X' corresponds to the quadrant examined.

In case the VA is less than 6/6, repeat the examination with a pinhole in front of the patient's eye being examined. Record the VA of the left eye, similarly, after occluding the right eye.

Note:
1. In case the VA is less than 6/60, check for projection of rays.
2. In case the patient is unable to comprehend/read, use the tumbling E-chart. The patient may be handed the

plastic Tumbling E optotype and asked to hold it, as seen on the chart. Alternatively, ask the patient to point to the direction in which the prongs of the E open.
3. In case of paucity of time, start from the 6/18 line, you can check for vision upwards in case acuity is lower, or ask the patient to read down in case vision is more than 6/18.

NON-CONTACT TONOMETRY

Indications: Routine examination

Materials: Non-contact tonometer, chair

Method (you may also refer to the users manual): Seat the patient comfortably in the chair and explain the procedure to the patient. You may demonstrate the airpuff and its noise to apprehensive patients, assuring them that nothing touches their eye, and the procedure is completely painless. Adjust the patient's height in the chin rest so that their outer canthus is aligned with the mark, ensure that the patient's forehead is well-apposed to the forehead rest.

Adjust the instrument height so that the light from the instrument objective shines in the center of the patient's pupil of the right eye. Raise the safety lock, ask the patient close their eyes and move the instrument forward until you see a donut-shaped bright area with a shadowed center on the patient's lid, then release the safety lock and make sure the instrument will not move any farther forward. Have the patient open their eyes and again center the light so that it shines in the center of the patient's pupil.

Ask the patient open his or her eyes wide (suggest that the patient "look surprised") and look right at the red dot or target. Your emphasis should now be on alignment and focusing of the dancing red target within the black reticule.

The target you see should have a white background with a central red dot. The red target should be moving, if it is stationary then you are either too close or too far away from the patient's eye. You should have one hand on the height adjustment with your index finger over the air puff control (trigger) and the other hand on the joy stick for lateral movements. Once the red dot is inside the reticule and in focus, depress the air puff trigger and you should get a reading on the display screen. This should be accompanied by a red light display located at the bottom of the display screen if the reading is accurate (NCT I only). The NCT II does not have this display light nor does it have an external fixation light.

Repeat the procedure twice for the same eye, and read the average of the three readings off the sceen.

Repeat the procedure for the left eye.

Interpretation: In case of intraocular pressure (IOP) records more than 21 mm Hg, please refer the patient for a Goldmann applanation tonometry.

Note:
1. First eye's measurements are often seen to be higher, and this is presumed to be due to the anxiousness of the patient and the co-contraction of the extraocular muscles to the feel and sound of the airpuff or the patient squinting.
2. The Icare TA01i may be used to provides a simple, easy, rapid, reliable, and accurate measurement of IOP, instead of NCT. The device probe may be sterilized between patients using isopropranolol.

ANTERIOR CHAMBER DEPTH

Indications: Routine examination, to rule out angle-closure glaucoma.

Material: Slit lamp

Method: Seat the patient on the slit lamp, looking straight ahead. Make a full length slit with low to medium illumination, and make sure that the angle between observation and illumination is 60°, magnification approximately 15×. Place optical section just inside limbus, and assess the anterior chamber (AC) depth, i.e., the gap from corneal endothelium to iris, assuming the corneal thickness to be 1 unit **(Fig. 1)**.

Van Herick grades of estimation of anterior chamber (AC) depth:

Grade	AC depth	Clinical interpretation	Corresponding angle in degrees
4	>½	Closure impossible	45–35
3	½–¼	Closure impossible	35–20
2	¼	Closure possible	20
1	<¼	Closure likely with full dilation	10 or less
0	Nil	Closed	0

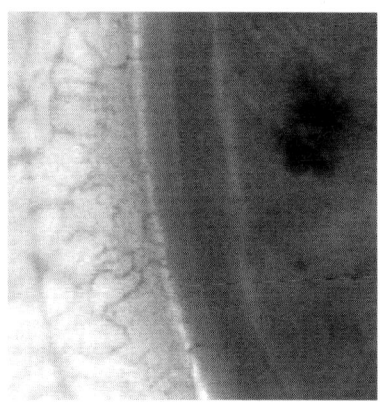

Fig. 1: Anterior chamber depth, van Herrick test.

Interpretation: All patients with a van Herick peripheral AC depth of 2 or less, must be referred for a gonioscopy.

SLIT-LAMP BIOMICROSCOPY: FUNDUS EXAMINATION 90 D LENS

Indications: Routine examination, to rule out retinal pathology

Materials: Slit lamp, 90 D lens

Method: Seat the patient on the slit lamp, looking straight ahead in a darkened room. Make a full length slit with low-to-medium illumination, and make sure that the angle between observation and illumination is 0°, magnification approximately 15×. Place optical section so as to achieve retroillumination and see the red fundal glow. Interpose the lens about 1 cm from the pupil, by resting your hands comfortably on the patient's forehead and holding the lens between your thumb and forefinger. Pull the slit lamp back until the aerial image of the fundus is focused. At an approximate distance of 1 cm, the lens comes into focus and after another 1 cm brings into sharp focus the fundal image between the lens and the slit-lamp objective. The fundus may then be examined by scanning across the field of view. Any measurements can be made by adjusting the slit-lamp beam height.

Interpretation:
- Note the cup to disc ratio and catagorize the disc into one of the following: Cup to disc ratio <0.3, 0.4–0.6 or >0.7. For screening purposes cup to disc ratio of >0.7 is considered to be abnormal.
- Any disc asymmetry of >0.2 is abnormal.

- The normal neuroretina rim thickness follows the pattern: Inferior, superior, nasal, temporal (the ISNT rule). Any deviation is considered abnormal, as is any pallor.
- Any hemorrhages on the disc must be noted and considered abnormal.

Note:
1. Follow the same procedure for all fundus lenses including the 66 D, 78 D, superfield lens, etc., in case a 90 D lens is not available.
2. Dilating the patient may facilitate the examination. Dilate all patients with diabetes, and suspected retinal pathologies.
3. Displacing the slit-lamp beam slightly off center, and reducing the beam width, both help reduce reflections.
4. The smartphone camera's coaxial flashlight and a handheld +15 D or +20 D lens may be used for disc documentation. The optical system records high-resolution digital disc images, which may be used for serial follow-up of these patients as well.

GOLDMANN APPLANATION TONOMETRY

Indications: It is to be performed if NCT > 21.

Materials: Slit-lamp, Goldmann applanation tonometer (GAT), fluorescein strips, local anesthetic.

Method: Explain to the patient the procedure, and the reasons for the same. Reassure the patient that his eye will be anesthetized, and that there will be no pain. Set the measuring drum on one (1 g, i.e., 10 mm Hg).

Align the white line on the probe carrier with the zero or 180 degree marker of the probe. If the corneal astigmatism is greater than 3 D, the measurement is made by aligning the red line on the probe carrier to the meridian of lower power. Use a wide open diffuse illumination, cobalt blue filter and 16× magnification with the light source 60–65° temporal to the probe. Ensure that the optical system and tonometer are offset by 5–10°.

Ensure that the patient is seated comfortably with the lateral canthus aligned with the canthal mark on the slit lamp, with the forehead pressing against the headrest. Instill a drop of local anesthetic, Proparacaine HCl or oxybuprivacaine, and gently touch the inferior fornix with a fluorescein strip. Alternatively, a drop of the commercially available fluorescein oxybuprivacaine combination may be used. Ask the patient to close his eyes and wipe off the excess with a tissue. Pre-align the eyes from outside the slit lamp, ask the patient to blink and then look straight ahead, with eyes open wide. Move the slit-lamp forward till you see a limbal glow, this signifies contact with the cornea.

See the mires through the slit lamp, mono-ocularly. If the mires are too wide, pull the slit lamp back and dry off the end of the probe and start over. Align the inner edges of the mires, till they just touch, by adjusting the setting of the measuring drum. In case of pulsations of the mires, the end point is the point with equal fluctuations on either side **(Fig. 2)**.

Examine the eyes to rule out any corneal staining, abrasion or edema. Lubricating drops may be prescribed as required for better patient comfort.

Interpretation: Note down your readings as the value read off the drum multiplied by ten, to arrive at the IOP

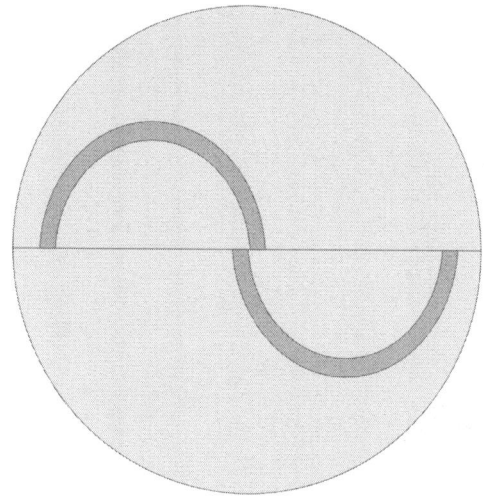

Fig. 2: Correct mire alignment in goldmann applanation tonometry (GAT).

in millimeters of mercury (mm Hg). A reading of >21 is considered abnormal for screening purposes.

GONIOSCOPY

Indications: To be performed in case van Herick ACD is Grade 2 or less.

Materials: Slit lamp, four-mirror goniolens, local anesthetic.

Method: Seat the patient comfortably at the slit lamp in a dark room. Instill local anesthetic drops. Ask the patient to look up, and gently put in the gonioscope. Ask the patient to look straight ahead. With the slit-lamp magnification at 10–25×, a fixed background illumination intensity and a small slit beam (2–3 mm) which does not traverse the pupil, observe the angle of the eye **(Figs. 3A and B)**. Note the structures visible, iris configuration,

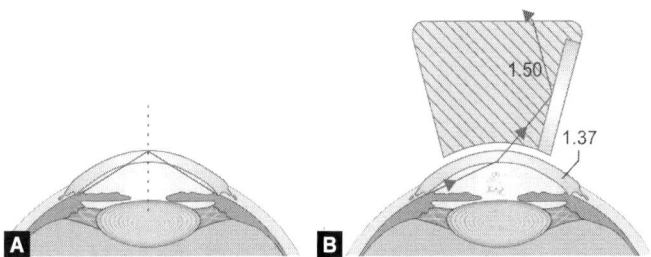

Figs. 3A and B: Principle of gonioscopy.

width of the recess, presence or absence of synechiae, pigment, pseudoexfoliation, and neovascularization in the angle. In case of angle closure, slight backward pressure (indentation) will help differentiate between appositional and synechial closure.

For detailed information about the method: http://www. gonioscopy.org.

Interpretation: The possibility of angle closure can be ruled out if the posterior trabecular meshwork is readily seen. The corneal wedge indicates the schwalbe's line, therefore if seen, implies that the angle is open. In case the angle is not seen to be open, the patient is to be referred for further evaluation.

# CHAPTER 14

Postscreening Follow-up

A referral mechanism to insure access to examination and treatment needs to be available in order to have an effective screening protocol. The efficacy measure of a screening program is not the total number of positive screens, but the actual case finding.

Therefore, it is imperative that the positive screens be followed up effectively in order to trace the definitive results of subsequent examinations.

The follow-up contact schedule is to be set-up for each screening unit individually, depending on the conditions on site. All postscreening follow-up exercises between 2 and 6 weeks following the screening camp should be considered a part of the valid screening protocol.

The following is the optimal postscreening contact protocol: Each patient with a positive screen result will receive a telephone call to see if they secured appointments. Phone calls are preferred as appointment and results can be confirmed immediately. In case where no phone or mail contact is possible, a caseworker/volunteer may visit the patient's home to ascertain if subsequent examinations have been performed. If not, the patient will be assisted in setting up their appointments at the medical facility. In case the test result is negative, the patient is advised to follow-up at the healthcare facility after a year. In case the patient has been diagnosed with glaucoma, a repeat contact is to be scheduled for 6 weeks after, to monitor compliance. Also, all first-degree relatives of the newly diagnosed case should be advised to visit the medical facility for a comprehensive eye check.

The second contact is to be scheduled for 2 weeks after the first contact to verify that the appointments scheduled have been kept, and the results of the definitive tests noted.

The subsequent course of action is the same as in case of the first contact: A negative result is to be counseled for subsequent follow-up, and a positive diagnosis monitored for compliance.

For follow through data, participants may also be asked to have healthcare providers fill out a brief form with a self-addressed stamped envelope to be mailed back to the screening program director for data gathering on diagnosis and treatment. However, the response rate is not expected to be adequate to enable data analysis, and therefore telephonic and/or face-to-face interviews are recommended in order to evaluate the efficacy of the screening program.

CHAPTER 15

Efficacy Measures

Given that each screening test has a known degree of error, a positive screen result is not a diagnosis. Each screening program requires a structure based on the distribution and determinants of disease. Identifying the target population and limiting the screening to the same, together with appropriate referrals and assisting with access to care is a measure of the effectiveness of the screening program.

Each screening program, especially one previously determined to not be a cost-effective exercise in general, must have an interim analysis built into its study protocol so that the same can justify continuing it in the specific population it is targeting.

EFFICACY MEASURES FOR THE SCREENING PROGRAM

- Yield is the number of new cases identified by the screening. The total number of positive screens that on further testing and evaluation are diagnosed as having glaucoma, will constitute the yield of the screening program.
- Market penetration is a measure of the amount of sales or adoption of a product or service compared to the total theoretical market for that product or service. In this case the total number of subjects from the target group screened, as a percentage of the total target population is a measure of utilization of the service provided.

- The number or percent of persons screened previously not screened or under care is a measure of the impact on community health.
- The most important index of efficacy of a screening program is the number or percent of persons referred and confirmed to have received care. It best measures the efficacy of the screening protocol in actually having a potential impact on disability limitation especially in those receiving treatment for previously unrecognized and asymptomatic glaucoma.

PERFORMANCE PARAMETERS TO BE EVALUATED FOR EACH OF THE SCREENING UNITS

- Response rate for each of the units and the regional disparity in the number of patients screened.
- Reasons for poor response, if any. Reasons for success, if any. Identifying both is essential for subsequent screening programs.
- Identification of lacunae and remedial measures for the same
- Revision of target group.

SUPERVISORS

- As the screening units will be functioning as semi-autonomous functionaries, each of the team leaders is responsible for an on-the-spot analysis of functioning, lacunae and remedies for the same.
- External supervision, including statistical overview of the case finding efficacy measures, must be performed at the end of one year from initiation of screening. This supervision will also be responsible for deciding if continuation of the screening program can be justified for the particular population.

TIMELINES

- Constant, on-the-spot, self-evaluation by the team leader.
- Interim analysis at one year to discuss the relative merits of further continuation of screening as against premature closure.
- Final analysis of efficacy measures at the end of two years of the screening program.

Appendix

WAIVER

Before participating in the screening program, you must understand and sign this document.

By signing this waiver, you also acknowledge that the check-up being offered to you is a screening for an eye disease called glaucoma, and is not a substitute for a comprehensive eye examination.

Glaucoma screening is recommended by health experts since glaucoma blindness is preventable. As most patients remain symptom free, it is important that you understand that regular, routine eye check-ups are very important.

The results of the screening will be provided and explained to you at the end of the procedure, with appropriate recommendations. In case you are identified as a glaucoma suspect, you will be advised to seek further management. In case there is no evidence of glaucoma at this point in time, you will be advised to continue having regular, routine eye check-ups over time.

In either case, you are advised to consult your eye specialist to better understand the results and implications of your screening.

By signing this document you also give permission for the use of the results of screening for your further treatment and follow-up, and also the informations obtained may be used for statistical analysis by the organizers of the camp for academic purposes, fully respecting your right to privacy.

This glaucoma screening program is being offered to you as part of glaucoma initiative, which assumes no risk or responsibility in connection with the procedures as part of a community glaucoma screening initiative by ------(insert Name of Organization),

Signature:
Name:
ID:
Contact:
Date/Place:

Signed in the presence of:

Signature:
Name:
Date/Place:

SCREENING FORM

Glaucoma Screening Initiative
Place:
Date:

Referred to:
Tel No.:
Patient ID No:

To be filled by patient/PMW

Name:

Date of Birth: Male ☐   Female ☐

Address: Tel No.:

Have you received any treatment for any eye disease?

     Yes ☐   No ☐

Have you had an eye injury, or any surgery on the eye?

     Yes ☐   No ☐

Are you suffering from:

	Yes	No	Not sure
Diabetes			
Hyper-tension			
Myopia			
Hyper-metropia			
Migraine			
Family h/o glaucoma			

Racial Origin:

Arab ☐   Asian ☐   African ☐

Hispanic ☐   European ☐

If IOP >22 → GAT

If VH <1/2 → Gonioscopy

To be completed by the doctor

	OD	OS
Visual acuity		
Visual acuity with pinhole		
IOP		
Van Herick		

Contd...

Contd...

Anterior segment: Cataract		
Pseudoex		
Infection		
Optic disc: C:D ratio		
NRR		
Hemorrhages		
Comments		

Recommendation:

☐ No suspicion of glaucoma → Routine annual check-up

☐ Glaucoma suspect → Refer to doctor/higher center for further evaluation

☐ Ophthalmic consultation for disorder other than glaucoma

Checked by [   ] on [   ]

Note: This is only a screening examination and is by no means a substitute for a comprehensive eye check-up.

POSTSCREENING FORM

To be completed by the paramedical workers

Patient ID No.: [ ]

Name:
Date of Birth: Male [ ]   Female [ ]
Address:
Tel No.:
Tested at:

Visit 1:
Diagnosis:
Advice:
Barriers to compliance:

Visit 2:
Compliance:
Side effects:
Barriers to compliance:

Comments:

Filled by: Name:
              Contact number:

SCREENING FEEDBACK FORM

Coordinator/Team Leader:

Contact number:

Date:

Location:

Doctor:

Technicians:

Volunteers:

Efficacy measures:

Total number of subjects screened:

Total number of positive screenings:

Total number of cataracts:

Comments:

Signature:
Date/Place:

Index

Page numbers followed by *f* refer to figure.

A

Acetazolamide 29
Adequate ambient light 31
Adequate emergency exits 32
Ancillary activities 10
Anterior chamber depth 37, 38*f*
Antibiotic ointment 30
Artificial intelligence, use of 5

B

Band-aids 30
Betadine 30
Blindness 1
Bombe 4

C

Cataract 15
Communication
    facilitating further 24
    skills 24
Community participation 26
Corneal
    endothelium 4
    staining 41
Cotton 30
Counselor station 29

D

Diabetic retinopathy 15
Dilated fundus examination 5
Disability limitation 47

E

E-chart reflected 9
Efficacy measures 46
Electrical points 31
Emergency medication kit 29
Equipment checklist 28
Error, degree of 46
Ethical clinical practice, general guidelines for 13
European Glaucoma Society 21
Eye 37, 41
    camp 9
    check-ups 49
    disease 49
    drops, antibiotic 29
    examination 49

F

Face-to-face interviews 45
First eye's measurements 37
Fluorescein oxybuprivacaine 41
Fundus examination 39
Furniture 31

G

Glaucoma 12, 16, 44, 49
    asymptomatic 47
    awareness
        development of 18
        week 17
    blindness 49

concerning 20
evidence of 49
family history of 1
implications of 21
problem of 20
screening for 1, 15, 49
   program 50
signs of secondary 4
stages of 3
symptoms of 15
vigilance for 19
Glaukomflecken 4
Goldmann applanation tonometry 37, 40, 42*f*
Gonioscopy 42
   principle of 43*f*

H

Healthcare
   facility 44
   professionals 12
Health-seeking behavior 21
Homatropine 29
Hygiene facilities 31
Hypermetropia 8

I

IEC material 20
Individual counseling 20
Individual units 23
Information, education and communication 18
Intraocular pressure 2
Iris
   rubeosis 4
   transillumination 4

L

Lacunae 6
   identification of 47
Laser peripheral iridotomy 1
Left eye 34, 35
Lens capsule 4
Light, perception of 35
Local medical practitioners 26

M

Manpower planning 10
Mass approach 18
Media 27
Monitoring and reporting 11
Mydriatic eye drops 29

N

Neovascular causes 4
Non-contact
   airpuff tonometer 3
   tonometry 36
Non-governmental organizations 26
Nurse worker 23

O

Ocular emergencies 13
Opportunistic screening 8
Optic disc hemorrhages 5
Optic nerve assessment 4

P

Paramedical worker 16, 23
Patient flow 33
Perkins applanation tonometer 3
Positive screen, criteria for 2

Index

Postscreening follow-up 44
Prescreening
  protocol 15
    implementation 10
Primary angle-closure disease 8
Program management timelines 10
Public glaucoma educational sessions 16
Pupil 36

R

Registration station 28

S

Schwalbe's line 43
Screening
  activity, location of 9
  community-based 8
  day 11
  feasibility of 7
  machinery 3
  program 9, 46
    efficacy measures for 46
Sectoral iris atrophy 4
Seeking permissions, general guidelines for 12
Slit-lamp 38
  anterior segment biomicroscopy 4
  biomicroscopy 2, 39
  station 28
Social media, role of 27
Standard operating procedures 34
Sterile bandages 30
Steroid eye drops 29
Swabs 30
Synechiae, posterior 4

T

Team 23
  desirable 24
  essential 23
  leader 25
Timolol eye drops 29
Tonometer 3
Tonometry station 28
Tropicamide 29

V

van Herrick test 38*f*
Vision 35
  preservation of 16
Visual acuity 6, 34
  station 28
Visual field testing 5
Voluntary organizations 26

W

Waiver 49
Whom to screen 8
World Glaucoma Association 21